How to Make Delicious Vegan Comfort Food Recipes

Creative Plant-Based Takes on Classic Crave-Worthy Meals

The Fix-It Guy

Copyright © The Fix-It Guy

This book is a work of non-fiction, depending on the genre. Any resemblance to actual persons, living or dead, or actual events is purely coincidental.

Table of Contents

Introduction

Welcome to the delicious world of plant-based comfort food! Are you ready to embark on a culinary journey that's not just good for your taste buds but also for your health and the planet? If so, buckle up because "How to Make Delicious Vegan Comfort Food Recipes" is about to become your new kitchen companion.

In a world that often associates comfort food with the cheesy, meaty, and downright indulgent, we're here to challenge the norms and prove that plant-based cuisine can be just as crave-worthy, if not more! Imagine sinking your teeth into a juicy BBQ Jackfruit Taco or savoring the creamy decadence of Mushroom Alfredo without a hint of guilt. Yes, we're talking about comfort food that not only satisfies your taste buds but also nourishes your body from the inside out.

But wait, there's more! This isn't your typical cookbook with bland salads and uninspiring tofu. No, we're bringing you a symphony of flavors, a celebration of textures, and a riot of colors, all in the name of creating meals that are not just good for you but downright irresistible.

Whether you're a seasoned vegan looking to spice up your repertoire or a curious carnivore dipping your toes into the world of plant-based goodness, this book has something for everyone. Expect mouthwatering recipes that will have you forgetting about meat and dairy in no time. We're not here to convert you; we're here to show you how darn delicious the plant-based life can be!

So, get ready to turn your kitchen into a haven of creativity, flavor, and joy. From appetizers that will steal the spotlight at any party to desserts that will make you the hero of family gatherings, we've got you covered.

Let the aroma of aromatic spices and the sizzle of wholesome ingredients be your guide on this exciting adventure. Are you ready to make your taste buds dance with delight? Then grab your apron, preheat that oven, and let's dive into the world of "How to Make Delicious Vegan Comfort Food Recipes: Creative Plant-Based Takes on Classic Crave-Worthy Meals." Your taste buds will thank you, and you might just find yourself wondering why you didn't make the switch sooner. Happy cooking!

Chapter 1

Kitchen Essentials

Must-Have Ingredients

Welcome to the heart of the action, my friend! In this chapter, we're diving into the essentials, the backbone of your plant-based culinary escapades. Think of these as your trusty sidekicks, your culinary comrades in arms. You may not be in a Michelin-starred kitchen, but trust me, these ingredients will make you feel like you are!

1. Fresh Produce Galore:

You want colors brighter than your favorite childhood crayon set. Start by choosing a rainbow of veggies, bell peppers, leafy greens, tomatoes, and more. Feeling adventurous? Add some exotic picks like kale or bok choy. Slice, dice, and let the vibrant hues take center stage.

Troubleshooting Tip: If your veggies look a bit sad, they've probably seen better days. Revive them by soaking in ice water for a quick refresh.

2. *Staples Straight from the Pantry:*

Your pantry is your secret weapon. Stock up on legumes like chickpeas and lentils, grains like quinoa and rice, and don't forget the magic of canned tomatoes. These staples are your canvas, waiting for your flavorful brushstrokes.

Troubleshooting Tip: Got a mountain of dried beans with no time to soak? No worries! Opt for canned ones – they're lifesavers.

3. *Herbs and Spices:*

Time to turn up the flavor! Gather garlic, ginger, basil, oregano, cumin, and whatever else makes your taste buds do a happy dance. Fresh or dried, these aromatic powerhouses will transform your creations.

Troubleshooting Tip: Spice rack looking a bit dusty? Revitalize your spices by giving them a quick sniff. If they don't smell vibrant, it's time for an upgrade.

4. *Nuts and Seeds:*

Welcome to the crunch party! Almonds, walnuts, chia seeds, and flaxseeds, these are your texture magicians. Sprinkle them on salads, toss them in smoothies, or snack on them solo.

Troubleshooting Tip: Can't find that bag of almonds you swore you bought? Check the depths of your pantry; they might be hiding behind the pasta.

5. Plant-Based Milk and Alternatives:

Milk a plant? Well, kind of. Explore almond milk, soy milk, coconut milk, the choices are as varied as your taste preferences. These will be your creamy accomplices in many a recipe.

Troubleshooting Tip: Curdled plant-based milk? It happens. Just stir in a bit of lemon juice or vinegar to bring it back to silky smoothness.

6. Condiments and Sauces:

Spice up your life with a collection of condiments. Soy sauce, hot sauce, tahini, and a jar of tomato sauce can be your best flavor buddies. They're like the cool kids at the flavor table.

Troubleshooting Tip: Forgot to grab ketchup for your fries? Try a dash of hot sauce mixed with a bit of sugar, makeshift ketchup, and a spicy one at that!

Remember, this is your kitchen adventure, so feel free to swap, mix, and match according to your taste buds' whims. These ingredients are just the starting point, the canvas for your culinary masterpiece.

Key Takeaway: Your plant-based journey begins with a well-stocked kitchen. So, raid that pantry, fill up the fridge, and get ready to create some veggie magic in the chapters to come!

Essential Cooking Tools

Now that you've got your ingredients ready to roll, let's talk about the unsung heroes of the kitchen – your trusty tools. It's like gearing up for a culinary adventure, and these gadgets are your culinary sidekicks. Batman has his utility belt, and you've got your kitchen arsenal!

1. Chef's Knife – Your Culinary Sword:
Invest in a good chef's knife. This isn't just a kitchen tool; it's an extension of your arm. Slice, dice, and chop with precision. Your veggies will thank you.

Troubleshooting Tip: Dull knife? Dull day. Sharpen that blade regularly, and watch your chopping game level up.

2. Cutting Boards – The Platform of Flavors:
Wooden or plastic, pick your poison. Just make sure it's spacious. No one wants a crowded cutting board – things might get dicey (pun intended).

Troubleshooting Tip: Caught a whiff of yesterday's onions on your cutting board? Sprinkle it with salt, scrub with a lemon half, and voilà, good as new.

3. Blender – The Smooth Operator:

Smoothies, soups, sauces, the blender does it all. Invest in a quality blender, and you'll wonder how you ever lived without it.

Troubleshooting Tip: Stuck with chunky soup when you wanted velvety smooth? Strain it through a sieve, and you'll be sipping elegance in no time.

4. Skillet and Saucepan – The Dynamic Duo:

Whether you're stir-frying veggies or simmering a savory sauce, a reliable skillet and saucepan are your kitchen dynamic duo.

Troubleshooting Tip: Sticky residue on your skillet? Sprinkle it with baking soda, add water, and let it simmer. The gunk will surrender.

5. Food Processor – The Time-Saver:

A food processor is like having a kitchen assistant. From nut butters to falafel mix, it's a multitasking marvel.

Troubleshooting Tip: Overworked hummus turning into a paste? Add a splash of water or olive oil to restore its creamy glory.

Tips for Efficient Vegan Cooking

1. Prep Like a Pro:

Before you start cooking, chop, measure, and organize. It's like having your own cooking show with everything prepped and ready to go.

Troubleshooting Tip: Ran out of counter space? Use large bowls or plates to hold prepped ingredients temporarily.

2. Master the Art of Batch Cooking:

Cook once, eat twice. Prepare larger quantities and freeze leftovers for those days when you just can't be bothered.

Troubleshooting Tip: Accidentally turned your pasta into mush? Embrace it as a pasta casserole, problem solved!

3. Embrace One-Pot Wonders:

Less mess, more flavor. Opt for one-pot recipes; they're a game-changer when you're not in the mood for a mountain of dishes.

Troubleshooting Tip: Rice sticking to the pot? Add a bit of oil before cooking or, better yet, invest in a non-stick pot.

4. Master the Art of Substitutions:
Out of an ingredient? Improvise! Swap in what you have, and let your creativity shine.

Troubleshooting Tip: No flaxseeds for that egg substitute? Chia seeds or applesauce work like magic.

5. Clean As You Go:
A cluttered kitchen is a stressed kitchen. Wash, wipe, and put away as you cook. It's like a victory lap after a successful dish.

Troubleshooting Tip: Stuck with burnt-on mess? Boil water in the pan, add baking soda, and let it sit. The gunk will surrender without a fight.

Key Takeaway: A well-equipped kitchen and savvy cooking tips are your secret weapons. Now, armed with these tools and tricks, you're ready to conquer the vegan culinary world. So, apron up, spatula in hand, and let the cooking adventures begin!

Chapter 2

Appetizers and Snacks

Guilt-Free Spinach Artichoke Dip

Ah, the gateway to any great meal, appetizers and snacks! In this chapter, we're kicking things off with a classic that's been reimagined into a guilt-free delight. Get ready to dive into the world of our tantalizing "Guilt-Free Spinach Artichoke Dip."

Let's Get Started:

Ingredients:
- 1 cup frozen spinach, thawed and drained
- 1 can artichoke hearts, chopped
- 1 cup vegan cream cheese
- 1 cup vegan mayonnaise
- 1 cup nutritional yeast
- 1/2 cup vegan grated Parmesan
- 2 cloves garlic, minced
- Salt and pepper to taste

Instructions:

1. Preheat and Prepare:
Preheat your oven to 375°F (190°C). Grease a baking dish, the anticipation is building!

Troubleshooting Tip: No baking dish? A cast-iron skillet works wonders.

2. Mixing Magic:
In a large bowl, mix the thawed and drained spinach, chopped artichoke hearts, vegan cream cheese, vegan mayo, nutritional yeast, vegan Parmesan, minced garlic, salt, and pepper. Give it a good stir, this is your creamy canvas.

Troubleshooting Tip: Too excited and forgot to thaw the spinach? Microwave it for a quick defrost.

3. Into the Oven:
Transfer your creamy concoction to the greased baking dish. Smooth the top like you're tucking it in for a cozy nap.

Troubleshooting Tip: Bubbling over? Place a baking sheet under the dish to catch any rebellious drips.

4. Bake to Perfection:

Pop it in the preheated oven for 25-30 minutes or until the edges are golden and the dip is bubbling with anticipation.

Troubleshooting Tip: Craving a golden crust? Broil for a couple of minutes, but keep an eye on it, things can go from golden to burnt real quick.

5. The Moment of Truth:

Remove from the oven and let it cool for a bit. The aroma is going to make your kitchen the most popular spot in the house.

Troubleshooting Tip: Overzealous dipping can lead to burnt tongues. Advise your guests to exercise caution.

6. Dive In with Dippers:

Grab your favorite dippers, tortilla chips, carrot sticks, or crispy baguette slices. Dip, scoop, and savor the guilt-free goodness.

Troubleshooting Tip: Ran out of chips? Veggie sticks are your crunchy sidekicks.

Key Takeaway:

This guilt-free Spinach Artichoke Dip is not just a crowd-pleaser; it's a sneak peek into the world of vegan delights. Creamy, savory, and bursting with flavor, this appetizer sets the tone for the culinary adventure ahead. So, gather your friends, grab those dippers, and let the dipping delight begin!

Buffalo Cauliflower Bites

Welcome to the flavor-packed world of Buffalo Cauliflower Bites, the snack that bites back! In this segment of our Appetizers and Snacks chapter, we're turning cauliflower into crispy, spicy morsels that will have your taste buds doing a happy dance.

Let's Get Started:

Ingredients:
- 1 medium-sized cauliflower, cut into florets
- 3/4 cup all-purpose flour
- 3/4 cup unsweetened almond milk
- 1 teaspoon garlic powder
- 1 teaspoon onion powder
- 1/2 teaspoon smoked paprika
- 1/2 teaspoon salt
- 1/4 teaspoon black pepper
- 1 cup buffalo hot sauce
- 2 tablespoons vegan butter, melted

Instructions:

1. Preheat for Perfection:
Preheat your oven to 450°F (230°C). Line a baking sheet with parchment paper, we're about to make some magic happen.

Troubleshooting Tip: Out of parchment paper? A lightly greased baking sheet works in a pinch.

2. Batter Up:

In a bowl, whisk together the flour, almond milk, garlic powder, onion powder, smoked paprika, salt, and black pepper. This is your flavor-packed batter.

Troubleshooting Tip: Batter too thick? Add a splash more almond milk for that perfect drizzle consistency.

3. Dip and Coat:

Dip each cauliflower floret into the batter, making sure it's fully coated. Place them on the prepared baking sheet with room to breathe, no crowded bites here.

Troubleshooting Tip: Fingers getting too messy? Embrace the mess; it's part of the fun!

4. Bake to Crispy Perfection:

Bake in the preheated oven for 20-25 minutes or until the cauliflower is golden and crispy. Flip them halfway through to ensure an even crunch.

Troubleshooting Tip: Bites not crispy enough? Give them an extra few minutes in the oven, and you'll have the crunch you crave.

5. Buffalo Bliss:

While the cauliflower is baking, mix the buffalo hot sauce and melted vegan butter in a bowl. Once the cauliflower is done, toss the bites in this spicy concoction until fully coated.

Troubleshooting Tip: Too hot to handle? A dollop of vegan ranch dressing on the side can cool things down.

6. Serve and Enjoy:

Arrange your buffalo cauliflower bites on a plate, perhaps with some celery sticks and vegan ranch on the side. It's time to indulge in spicy, tangy goodness.

Troubleshooting Tip: Forgot the celery? Carrot sticks are crunchy substitutes.

Key Takeaway:

Buffalo Cauliflower Bites are the game-day snack you never knew you needed. Spicy, crispy, and downright addictive, they're a testament to the wonders of plant-based eating. So, whether you're a spice enthusiast or a cauliflower skeptic, get ready to be converted, one bite at a time.

Creamy Avocado Hummus

Now, let's switch gears and dive into the world of Creamy Avocado Hummus, a green twist on the classic dip. Get ready to elevate your snacking experience with a blend of chickpeas and the almighty avocado.

Let's Get Started:

Ingredients:
- 1 can (15 oz) chickpeas, drained and rinsed
- 2 ripe avocados, peeled and pitted
- 3 tablespoons tahini
- 2 cloves garlic, minced
- 1/4 cup fresh cilantro or parsley, chopped
- Juice of 1 lemon
- 2 tablespoons olive oil
- Salt and pepper to taste

Instructions:

1. Blend, Baby, Blend:
In a food processor, combine the chickpeas, avocados, tahini, minced garlic, cilantro or parsley, lemon juice, and olive oil. Blend until smooth – this is your green dream in the making.

Troubleshooting Tip: Hummus too thick? Add a bit more olive oil or a splash of water for that perfect dip consistency.

2. Season to Perfection:

Season your avocado hummus with salt and pepper, adjusting to your taste preferences. Give it a final whirl in the food processor to ensure everything is beautifully incorporated.

Troubleshooting Tip: Hummus too bland? A pinch of cumin or a dash of paprika can add that extra oomph.

3. Chill and Relax:

Transfer your creamy creation into a bowl and refrigerate for at least 30 minutes. This gives the flavors a chance to mingle and dance.

Troubleshooting Tip: Impatiently hungry? It's okay; you can dive in immediately, but the flavors get even better with time.

4. Serve with Style:

When you're ready to indulge, serve your Creamy Avocado Hummus with a drizzle of olive oil, a sprinkle of chopped cilantro or parsley, and perhaps a few cherry tomatoes on top. Break out the pita chips, veggie sticks, or your favorite crackers, it's snack time!

Troubleshooting Tip: Ran out of crackers? Toasted bread or pretzels work wonders.

Key Takeaway:

Creamy Avocado Hummus is not just a dip; it's a celebration of green goodness. Creamy, zesty, and with a hint of herbaceous freshness, this dip is a versatile star. Whether you're hosting a gathering or simply treating yourself, let the creamy allure of avocado hummus take center stage.

Enjoy the snack journey, my friend! These recipes are more than just bites; they're little moments of culinary joy. Happy snacking!

Chapter 3

Hearty Soups and Stews

Classic Tomato Basil Soup

Now, let's cozy up to the warmth of Chapter 3, a haven for comfort seekers, the realm of hearty soups and stews. In this chapter, we're turning the spotlight onto a timeless favorite: the "Classic Tomato Basil Soup."

Ingredients:

- 2 cans (28 oz each) whole peeled tomatoes
- 1/4 cup olive oil
- 1 large onion, chopped
- 4 cloves garlic, minced
- 4 cups vegetable broth
- 1/2 cup fresh basil, chopped
- 1 teaspoon sugar
- Salt and pepper to taste
- 1/2 cup vegan cream (optional, for extra creaminess)

Instructions:

1. Tomato Tango:
Start by opening those cans of whole peeled tomatoes. Don't drain them, we want all that tomatoey goodness. Crush the tomatoes with your hands (it's therapeutic) or use a spoon. Set aside.

Troubleshooting Tip: Can't find whole tomatoes? Diced ones work in a pinch.

2. Sauté Symphony:
In a large pot, heat the olive oil over medium heat. Add the chopped onions and sauté until they're dancing in golden glory. Toss in the minced garlic and let the aroma serenade your senses.

Troubleshooting Tip: Onion-induced tears? Chew gum while chopping, it helps.

3. Tomato Ballet:
Introduce those crushed tomatoes to the pot. Let them twirl with the onions and garlic. Add a pinch of sugar to balance the acidity. Stir like you're conducting a symphony.

Troubleshooting Tip: Too acidic? Counteract with a bit more sugar or a splash of balsamic vinegar.

4. Broth Ballet:

Pour in the vegetable broth, letting it pirouette into the mix. Season generously with salt and pepper. Bring the ensemble to a gentle boil, then reduce the heat and let it simmer.

Troubleshooting Tip: Too salty? Dilute with a bit of water or low-sodium broth.

5. Basil Waltz:

While your soup orchestra is simmering away, add the chopped fresh basil. Let it pirouette into the mix, infusing its aromatic magic.

Troubleshooting Tip: Out of fresh basil? Dried basil can step in, just use less as it's more potent.

6. Creamy Crescendo (Optional):

Want to elevate the creaminess? Pour in the vegan cream, stirring gently. This is the crescendo, the moment of pure indulgence.

Troubleshooting Tip: Curdling cream? Remove the soup from heat and stir slowly. Or, use an immersion blender for a smoother texture.

7. Soul-Soothing Simmer:

Let the soup simmer for at least 20-30 minutes. Longer if you can resist the temptation. This simmering symphony enhances the flavors, turning them into a harmony of comfort.

Troubleshooting Tip: Impatient taste buds? It's hard, but the longer it simmers, the richer the flavors.

8. Serve and Savor:

Ladle this soul-warming elixir into bowls. Top with a sprinkle of fresh basil or a swirl of vegan cream. Each spoonful is a journey into the heart of comfort.

Troubleshooting Tip: Forgot the toppings? A drizzle of olive oil or a pinch of black pepper can save the day.

Key Takeaway:

The Classic Tomato Basil Soup is more than just a recipe; it's a celebration of simplicity and comfort. With every spoonful, you're tasting the timeless embrace of a familiar favorite. So, get that ladle ready, cozy up with a bowl, and let the warmth of this classic soup wrap around you like a familiar hug. Enjoy!

Lentil and Vegetable Stew

In this delightful chapter, we're venturing further into the heartiness of soups and stews, and two stars are about to take center stage: the "Lentil and Vegetable Stew" and the "Coconut Curry Butternut Squash Soup."

Ingredients:

- 1 cup dried green or brown lentils
- 1 large onion, diced
- 3 carrots, sliced
- 3 celery stalks, chopped
- 4 cloves garlic, minced
- 1 can (14 oz) diced tomatoes
- 1 can (14 oz) tomato sauce
- 6 cups vegetable broth
- 1 teaspoon ground cumin
- 1 teaspoon paprika
- 1 teaspoon dried thyme
- Salt and pepper to taste
- 2 cups kale or spinach, chopped
- Lemon wedges for serving

Instructions:

1. Lentil Love Affair:

Begin by rinsing the lentils under cold water. Set aside. This is the start of a beautiful relationship.

Troubleshooting Tip: Lentils sticking to the pot? Stir occasionally, and add a bit of oil if needed.

2. Sauté Symphony:

In a large pot, sauté the diced onion, carrots, celery, and minced garlic until they're a golden dream team.

Troubleshooting Tip: Browning too quickly? Lower the heat and stir more often.

3. Tomato Tango:

Add the diced tomatoes and tomato sauce to the pot. Let them join the veggie party, infusing their rich flavors.

Troubleshooting Tip: Too acidic? Balance with a pinch of sugar or a drizzle of balsamic vinegar.

4. Lentil Embrace:

Introduce the rinsed lentils to the mix. Pour in the vegetable broth, and season with ground cumin, paprika, dried thyme, salt, and pepper. Let this flavorful fusion simmer.

Troubleshooting Tip: Lentils still firm after simmering? Patience is key, they need time to soften.

5. *Greens Galore:*

When the lentils are tender, add the chopped kale or spinach. This is the final flourish, adding a burst of color and nutrients.

Troubleshooting Tip: Overwhelmed by the green avalanche? Start with less and add more if needed.

6. *Lemon Lift:*

Squeeze fresh lemon juice over each serving just before diving in. The citrusy zing elevates the flavors to a whole new level.

Troubleshooting Tip: No fresh lemons? A dash of apple cider vinegar can bring that acidity.

Key Takeaway:

The Lentil and Vegetable Stew isn't just a stew; it's a wholesome, nutrient-packed embrace. With each spoonful, you're nourishing both body and soul. So, ladle up, savor the goodness, and revel in the joy of a comforting bowl.

Coconut Curry Butternut Squash Soup

Ingredients:

- 1 medium butternut squash, peeled and diced
- 1 onion, chopped
- 3 cloves garlic, minced
- 1 tablespoon curry powder
- 1 teaspoon ground cumin
- 1 teaspoon ground coriander
- 1/2 teaspoon red pepper flakes (adjust for spice preference)
- 1 can (14 oz) coconut milk
- 4 cups vegetable broth
- 1 tablespoon coconut oil
- Salt and pepper to taste
- Fresh cilantro for garnish

Instructions:

1. Butternut Ballet:

Start by peeling and dicing the butternut squash. This might feel like a workout, but trust me, the soup is worth it.

Troubleshooting Tip: Struggling with the squash? Microwave it for a minute to soften the skin.

2. Sauté Serenade:

In a large pot, sauté the chopped onion and minced garlic in coconut oil until they're golden and fragrant. This is the aromatic prelude to your curry masterpiece.

Troubleshooting Tip: Burning garlic alert? Lower the heat and stir swiftly, burnt garlic is bitter.

3. Curry Canvas:

Sprinkle in the curry powder, ground cumin, ground coriander, and red pepper flakes. Let the spices create a flavorful canvas.

Troubleshooting Tip: Not a fan of spice? Tone down the red pepper flakes or omit them entirely.

4. Squash Symphony:

Add the diced butternut squash to the pot. Coat it in the fragrant spice mixture, letting each cube soak up the flavors.

Troubleshooting Tip: Squash sticking to the pot? Add a splash of vegetable broth to deglaze.

5. Creamy Crescendo:

Pour in the coconut milk and vegetable broth. Bring the symphony to a gentle boil, then reduce the heat and let it simmer until the squash is tender.

Troubleshooting Tip: Curdled coconut milk? Fear not, an immersion blender can smooth out the texture.

6. Blitz and Bliss:

Use an immersion blender to blitz the soup into velvety smoothness. If you don't have an immersion blender, transfer the soup to a blender in batches.

Troubleshooting Tip: Too thick? Add more vegetable broth until it reaches your desired consistency.

7. Season and Serve:

Season the soup with salt and pepper to taste. Ladle into bowls, garnish with fresh cilantro, and behold the creamy curry magic.

Troubleshooting Tip: Too salty? A squeeze of lime can balance the flavors.

Key Takeaway:

The Coconut Curry Butternut Squash Soup is a dance of creaminess and spice. Each spoonful is a journey through the warm, aromatic richness of a well-spiced bowl. So, savor the velvety goodness, and let this soup be your passport to cozy evenings and contented smiles.

Chapter 4

Satisfying Salads

Caesar Salad with Cashew Caesar Dressing

Ah, the crisp crunch of fresh greens and the tantalizing embrace of flavorful dressings, welcome to the vibrant world of satisfying salads. In this chapter, we're shining the spotlight on a classic with a plant-based twist: the "Caesar Salad with Cashew Caesar Dressing."

Ingredients:

For the Salad:
- 1 head of romaine lettuce, chopped
- 1 cup cherry tomatoes, halved
- 1 cup croutons (store-bought or homemade)
- 1/4 cup vegan Parmesan cheese, grated
- 1/4 cup capers (optional for that briny kick)

For the Cashew Caesar Dressing:
- 1 cup raw cashews, soaked for at least 2 hours
- 1/4 cup nutritional yeast
- 2 cloves garlic, minced

- 2 tablespoons Dijon mustard
- 2 tablespoons capers, drained
- 1 tablespoon vegan Worcestershire sauce
- Juice of 1 lemon
- 1/2 cup water
- Salt and pepper to taste

Instructions:

1. Cashew Soak and Dream:

Begin by soaking the raw cashews for at least 2 hours. This softens them up, making them dreamy for blending into the dressing.

Troubleshooting Tip: Forgot to soak? Quick-soak in hot water for 15 minutes.

2. Dress to Impress:

In a blender, combine the soaked cashews, nutritional yeast, minced garlic, Dijon mustard, capers, vegan Worcestershire sauce, lemon juice, water, salt, and pepper. Blend until you achieve a creamy, luscious dressing.

Troubleshooting Tip: Too thick? Add a bit more water, one tablespoon at a time, until it reaches the desired consistency.

3. Salad Symphony:

In a large bowl, toss the chopped romaine lettuce, halved cherry tomatoes, croutons, vegan Parmesan cheese, and capers (if using). This is the canvas for your Caesar masterpiece.

Troubleshooting Tip: Soggy croutons? Toast them in a dry pan for a crisp revival.

4. Dress for Success:

Drizzle that velvety Cashew Caesar Dressing over the salad. Coat each leaf and crouton generously – don't be shy!

Troubleshooting Tip: Want an extra kick? Add a pinch of black pepper or a sprinkle of red pepper flakes.

5. Toss and Turn:

Gently toss the salad, ensuring every leaf is caressed by the creamy dressing. It's a toss-and-turn dance of flavors.

Troubleshooting Tip: Salad unevenly dressed? Drizzle a bit more dressing strategically and toss again.

6. Plate and Garnish:

Plate the Caesar Salad, garnishing with extra croutons, a sprinkle of vegan Parmesan, and a flourish of capers. This is your chance to make it Instagram-worthy!

Troubleshooting Tip: Too pretty to eat? Capture the moment with a quick snapshot.

7. Serve and Savor:

Dive into the world of flavors with a forkful of your homemade Caesar Salad. Let the crisp lettuce, tangy dressing, and crunchy croutons dance on your taste buds.

Troubleshooting Tip: Dressing leftovers? It doubles as a delightful dip for veggies or a sandwich spread.

Key Takeaway:

The Caesar Salad with Cashew Caesar Dressing is a testament to the fact that salads can be hearty, satisfying, and utterly delicious. So, toss away the notion that salads are just for rabbits – this one's a meal fit for a king or queen. Enjoy the vibrant, crunchy medley, and revel in the creamy delight of a well-dressed salad.

Quinoa and Roasted Vegetable Salad

In this chapter, we're delving into two more culinary gems that redefine the salad game, the "Quinoa and Roasted Vegetable Salad" and the "Southwestern Black Bean Salad."

Ingredients:

For the Salad:
- 1 cup quinoa, rinsed
- 2 cups mixed vegetables (bell peppers, cherry tomatoes, zucchini), chopped
- 1 red onion, thinly sliced
- 1 cup cucumber, diced
- 1/2 cup fresh parsley, chopped
- 1/4 cup feta cheese, crumbled (optional for a tangy kick)
- 1/4 cup almonds, sliced and toasted

For the Lemon Vinaigrette:
- 1/4 cup olive oil
- Juice of 1 lemon
- 1 teaspoon Dijon mustard
- 1 clove garlic, minced
- Salt and pepper to taste

Instructions:

1. Quinoa Magic:

Start by cooking the quinoa. Combine 1 cup of rinsed quinoa with 2 cups of water in a pot. Bring to a boil, then reduce heat, cover, and simmer for about 15 minutes or until the quinoa is cooked and water is absorbed.

Troubleshooting Tip: Sticky quinoa? Fluff it with a fork and let it cool before assembling the salad.

2. Veggie Extravaganza:

While the quinoa is cooking, toss the chopped mixed vegetables in olive oil, salt, and pepper. Roast them in the oven until they're golden and caramelized.

Troubleshooting Tip: Veggies sticking to the pan? Use parchment paper for easy cleanup.

3. Assemble the Symphony:

In a large bowl, combine the cooked quinoa, roasted vegetables, thinly sliced red onion, diced cucumber, chopped parsley, crumbled feta (if using), and sliced toasted almonds. This is a symphony of textures and flavors.

Troubleshooting Tip: Overwhelmed by chopping? Prep veggies in advance or use a food processor for quick chopping.

4. Dress to Impress:

In a small bowl, whisk together olive oil, lemon juice, Dijon mustard, minced garlic, salt, and pepper. This zesty concoction is your lemon vinaigrette.

Troubleshooting Tip: Too tangy? Add a touch of honey or maple syrup to balance the acidity.

5. Drizzle and Toss:

Drizzle the lemon vinaigrette over the salad and toss gently to coat. Each quinoa grain and vegetable should glisten with the citrusy goodness.

Troubleshooting Tip: Not a fan of lemon? Try balsamic vinaigrette for a different twist.

6. Serve and Sprinkle:

Plate your Quinoa and Roasted Vegetable Salad and sprinkle with extra feta, parsley, and toasted almonds for a finishing touch. Your masterpiece is ready to be savored.

Troubleshooting Tip: Guests running late? Hold off on adding the dressing until serving time to keep things fresh.

Southwestern Black Bean Salad

Ingredients:
- 2 cans (15 oz each) black beans, drained and rinsed
- 1 cup corn kernels (fresh, frozen, or canned)
- 1 red bell pepper, diced
- 1 orange or yellow bell pepper, diced
- 1 cup cherry tomatoes, halved
- 1/2 red onion, finely chopped
- 1 avocado, diced
- 1/4 cup fresh cilantro, chopped

For the Lime Cilantro Dressing:
- 1/4 cup olive oil
- Juice of 2 limes
- 1 teaspoon ground cumin
- 1/2 teaspoon chili powder
- 1 clove garlic, minced
- Salt and pepper to taste

Instructions:

1. Black Bean Fiesta:
In a large bowl, combine the black beans, corn kernels, diced red and yellow bell peppers, halved cherry tomatoes, finely chopped red onion, diced avocado, and chopped cilantro. It's a colorful fiesta in the making.

Troubleshooting Tip: Avocado too ripe? Mash it and turn it into a creamy dressing.

2. Whisk the Zest:

In a small bowl, whisk together olive oil, lime juice, ground cumin, chili powder, minced garlic, salt, and pepper. This zesty potion is your Lime Cilantro Dressing.

Troubleshooting Tip: Too tangy? A pinch of sugar or honey can mellow out the acidity.

3. Dress the Dance:

Drizzle the Lime Cilantro Dressing over the salad, and toss gently to ensure every bean and veggie is coated in the zesty goodness. The dressing is the rhythm that ties the flavors together.

Troubleshooting Tip: Want a smoky twist? Add a touch of smoked paprika to the dressing.

4. Chill and Infuse:

Let the Southwestern Black Bean Salad chill in the fridge for at least 30 minutes. This allows the flavors to mingle and dance together, reaching a crescendo of taste.

Troubleshooting Tip: Hungry and can't wait? Dive in right away, but the flavors intensify with time.

5. Serve and Garnish:

Plate your Southwestern masterpiece and garnish with extra cilantro. The vibrant colors and bold flavors are a feast for the eyes and the taste buds.

Troubleshooting Tip: Running low on cilantro? Fresh parsley can step in with its own burst of freshness.

Key Takeaway:

The Southwestern Black Bean Salad is not just a salad; it's a fiesta on your plate. Bursting with colors, textures, and bold flavors, each bite is a celebration of the vibrant ingredients. So, dish up, enjoy the party in your mouth, and revel in the fusion of southwestern flair and fresh goodness.

Chapter 5

Comforting Pasta Dishes

Creamy Mushroom Alfredo

As we venture into the realm of comforting pasta dishes, get ready for a culinary hug that transcends time and tradition. In this chapter, our spotlight falls on the "Creamy Mushroom Alfredo", a velvety symphony of pasta perfection.

Ingredients:

- 16 oz fettuccine pasta
- tablespoons olive oil
- 1 pound cremini or white mushrooms, sliced
- 4 cloves garlic, minced
- 1 cup vegetable broth
- 1 cup unsweetened almond milk (or any plant-based milk)
- 1 cup raw cashews, soaked for at least 2 hours
- 1/2 cup nutritional yeast
- Juice of 1 lemon
- Salt and pepper to taste
- Fresh parsley, chopped, for garnish

Instructions:

1. Pasta Prelude:

Cook the fettuccine pasta according to the package instructions. Drain and set aside. This is the canvas for your creamy masterpiece.

Troubleshooting Tip: Sticky pasta strands? A drizzle of olive oil after draining prevents clumping.

2. Mushroom Magic:

In a large skillet, heat olive oil over medium heat. Add the sliced mushrooms and sauté until they release their moisture and turn golden brown. The aroma is your cue, mushrooms are magic in the making.

Troubleshooting Tip: Crowded skillet? Sauté mushrooms in batches for that golden sear.

3. Garlic Serenade:

Introduce minced garlic to the golden mushrooms. Let them dance together for a minute until the fragrance fills the kitchen. This is the aromatic prelude to your Alfredo symphony.

Troubleshooting Tip: Burnt garlic alert? Lower the heat and stir swiftly, burnt garlic is bitter.

4. Cashew Cream Crescendo:

In a blender, combine soaked cashews, vegetable broth, almond milk, nutritional yeast, lemon juice, salt, and pepper. Blend until you achieve a smooth, creamy consistency. This cashew cream is the star of your Alfredo show.

Troubleshooting Tip: Cashew cream too thick? Add a bit more vegetable broth to reach the desired creaminess.

5. Alfredo Harmony:

Pour the cashew cream over the sautéed mushrooms and garlic in the skillet. Stir gently, letting the flavors harmonize into a luxurious Alfredo sauce. Simmer for a few minutes until it thickens slightly.

Troubleshooting Tip: Sauce too thin? Simmer a bit longer to reach your desired consistency.

6. Pasta and Sauce Ballet:

Add the cooked fettuccine pasta to the skillet, tossing it gently in the velvety mushroom Alfredo sauce. Every strand should be coated in this creamy embrace.

Troubleshooting Tip: Uneven coating? Use tongs to ensure every pasta strand gets its fair share of sauce.

7. *Plate and Garnish:*

Plate your Creamy Mushroom Alfredo, and garnish with a sprinkle of fresh chopped parsley. This touch of green adds a burst of freshness to the richness of the dish.

Troubleshooting Tip: Out of parsley? A drizzle of olive oil or a pinch of nutritional yeast can also enhance the presentation.

8. *Serve and Savor:*

Dive into the comforting indulgence of your Creamy Mushroom Alfredo. Each bite is a journey into the heart of pasta perfection, where creamy textures and umami flavors unite.

Troubleshooting Tip: Leftovers? Reheat gently with a splash of plant-based milk for that fresh-from-the-stove creaminess.

Key Takeaway:

The Creamy Mushroom Alfredo is more than a pasta dish; it's a celebration of velvety richness and earthy flavors. So, swirl your fork, savor the comforting embrace, and let this dish transport you to a world where every bite is a moment of pure indulgence.

Eggplant Parmesan with Cashew Cheese

In this chapter of comforting pasta dishes, we're diving into two classics with a plant-based twist, "Eggplant Parmesan with Cashew Cheese" and "Spaghetti Bolognese with Lentil Meatballs."

Ingredients:

For the Eggplant Parmesan:
- 2 large eggplants, sliced into rounds
- 1 cup breadcrumbs
- 1 cup marinara sauce
- 1 cup vegan mozzarella cheese, shredded
- Olive oil for drizzling
- Fresh basil, chopped, for garnish

For the Cashew Cheese:
- 1 cup raw cashews, soaked for at least 2 hours
- 1/4 cup nutritional yeast
- Juice of 1 lemon
- 1 clove garlic, minced
- Salt and pepper to taste

Instructions:

1. Eggplant Elegance:
Preheat your oven to 375°F (190°C). Place eggplant rounds on a baking sheet, drizzle with olive oil, and bake until they're golden and tender. This is the foundation of your Eggplant Parmesan.

Troubleshooting Tip: Sticky eggplant slices? Ensure they're not crowded on the baking sheet for an even bake.

2. Cashew Cheese Creation:
In a blender, combine soaked cashews, nutritional yeast, lemon juice, minced garlic, salt, and pepper. Blend until you achieve a creamy consistency. This cashew cheese is your dairy-free delight.

Troubleshooting Tip: Too thick? Add water, one tablespoon at a time, until it reaches your desired creaminess.

3. Layer and Repeat:
In a baking dish, layer the baked eggplant rounds with marinara sauce, vegan mozzarella, and a dollop of cashew cheese. Repeat until you've built a delicious tower of layers.

Troubleshooting Tip: Not a fan of marinara? Pesto or a simple tomato sauce works wonders too.

4. Bake to Melty Perfection:
Pop the dish into the preheated oven and bake until the cheese is melty and golden. The aroma wafting through your kitchen is the signal that your Eggplant Parmesan is ready to shine.

Troubleshooting Tip: Cheese not melting evenly? Cover with foil and bake a bit longer.

5. Garnish and Serve:
Sprinkle chopped fresh basil over your bubbly creation. The contrast of green adds a burst of freshness. Serve your Eggplant Parmesan with a side of joy.

Troubleshooting Tip: Basil not your style? Oregano or parsley can also bring a lovely herbaceous touch.

6. Savor the Layers:
Dive into your layers of eggplant goodness. Each forkful is a journey through the creamy cashew cheese, savory marinara, and tender eggplant. Buon Appetito!

Troubleshooting Tip: Leftovers? Reheat in the oven for a crispy top layer.

Key Takeaway:
The Eggplant Parmesan with Cashew Cheese is a testament to the fact that plant-based can be indulgent. So, slice, layer, and savor the richness of Italian flavors without compromising on taste.

Spaghetti Bolognese with Lentil Meatballs

Ingredients:

For the Lentil Meatballs:
- 1 cup dry green or brown lentils, cooked
- 1/2 cup breadcrumbs
- 1/4 cup vegan Parmesan cheese, grated
- 1 flax egg (1 tablespoon flaxseed meal + 3 tablespoons water)
- 1 teaspoon Italian seasoning
- Salt and pepper to taste
- Olive oil for baking

For the Spaghetti Bolognese:
- 16 oz spaghetti pasta
- 1 tablespoon olive oil
- 1 onion, finely chopped
- 2 carrots, grated
- 2 celery stalks, finely chopped
- 4 cloves garlic, minced
- 1 can (28 oz) crushed tomatoes
- 1 teaspoon dried oregano
- 1 teaspoon dried basil
- Salt and pepper to taste
- Fresh parsley, chopped, for garnish

Instructions:

1. Lentil Meatball Prep:
Preheat your oven to 375°F (190°C). In a bowl, combine cooked lentils, breadcrumbs, vegan Parmesan, flax egg, Italian seasoning, salt, and pepper. Roll this mixture into bite-sized lentil meatballs.

Troubleshooting Tip: Mixture too wet? Add more breadcrumbs; too dry? Add a splash of water.

2. Bake to Perfection:
Place the lentil meatballs on a baking sheet lined with parchment paper. Drizzle with olive oil and bake until they're golden and firm. This is the foundation of your Bolognese feast.

Troubleshooting Tip: Sticking to the pan? Parchment paper is your non-stick superhero.

3. Bolognese Symphony:
Cook the spaghetti according to the package instructions. In a separate pot, heat olive oil and sauté finely chopped onion, grated carrots, chopped celery, and minced garlic until they're softened and fragrant.

Troubleshooting Tip: Burning veggies? Lower the heat and stir more often.

4. *Tomato Tango:*

Add crushed tomatoes, dried oregano, dried basil, salt, and pepper to the sautéed veggies. Let this tomatoey symphony simmer until it's thick and flavorful.

Troubleshooting Tip: Too tangy? A pinch of sugar or a splash of balsamic vinegar can balance the acidity.

5. *Meatball Marriage:*

Gently fold your baked lentil meatballs into the simmering Bolognese sauce. Let them mingle and absorb the rich flavors.

Troubleshooting Tip: Sauce too thick? Add a bit of vegetable broth to reach your desired consistency.

6. *Serve and Garnish:*

Plate your spaghetti and ladle the lentil Bolognese over the top. Garnish with a sprinkle of chopped fresh parsley. This dash of green adds a burst of freshness to your hearty feast.

Troubleshooting Tip: Out of fresh parsley? A drizzle of olive oil or a pinch of nutritional yeast can also enhance the presentation.

7. *Taste the Heartiness:*

Twirl your fork and savor the hearty goodness of your Spaghetti Bolognese with Lentil Meatballs. Each bite is a journey through savory lentil bliss, tangled with perfectly cooked pasta.

Troubleshooting Tip: Lentil meatballs falling apart? Be gentle when stirring into the sauce, or let them firm up a bit more in the oven.

Key Takeaway:

The Spaghetti Bolognese with Lentil Meatballs is a celebration of Italian comfort, reimagined with plant-based flair. So, twirl those noodles, savor

Chapter 6

Creative Main Courses

BBQ Jackfruit Tacos

As we dive into the realm of creative main courses, get ready for a culinary adventure that pushes the boundaries of flavor. In this chapter, our spotlight is on "BBQ Jackfruit Tacos" a plant-based twist that brings bold and smoky barbecue goodness to your taco night.

Ingredients:

For the BBQ Jackfruit:
- 2 cans (20 oz each) young green jackfruit in brine, drained and shredded
- 1 cup barbecue sauce (choose your favorite
- 1 tablespoon olive oil
- 1 teaspoon smoked paprika
- 1 teaspoon garlic powder
- 1/2 teaspoon cumin
- Salt and pepper to taste

For the Tacos:
- 8 small corn or flour tortillas
- 1 cup purple cabbage, thinly sliced
- 1 avocado, sliced
- 1/2 cup fresh cilantro, chopped
- 1 lime, cut into wedges

Instructions:

1. Jackfruit Transformation:

Drain and shred the young green jackfruit using your hands or forks. In a skillet, heat olive oil over medium heat and add the shredded jackfruit. Sauté for a few minutes until it starts to brown.

Troubleshooting Tip: Jackfruit sticking to the pan? Add a bit more oil or reduce the heat.

2. Spice Infusion:

Sprinkle smoked paprika, garlic powder, cumin, salt, and pepper over the jackfruit. Stir to coat each strand with the smoky goodness.

Troubleshooting Tip: Not a fan of spice? Adjust the smoked paprika to your liking.

3. BBQ Bath:

Pour the barbecue sauce over the seasoned jackfruit. Stir well, ensuring every piece gets drenched in the savory barbecue bath. Let it simmer until the jackfruit absorbs the flavors and becomes tender.

Troubleshooting Tip: Too saucy? Simmer a bit longer to reduce the sauce.

4. Tortilla Toasting:

While the jackfruit is simmering, heat the tortillas on a griddle or in a dry skillet until they're warm and slightly toasted. This step enhances the taco experience.

Troubleshooting Tip: Tortillas too dry? Cover them with a damp cloth while warming.

5. Taco Assembly Line:

Set up your taco assembly line. Place a generous spoonful of the BBQ jackfruit onto each tortilla. Top it with thinly sliced purple cabbage, avocado slices, and a sprinkle of fresh cilantro.

Troubleshooting Tip: Avocado not ripe? A squeeze of lime can add that citrusy kick.

6. Garnish and Serve:

Garnish your BBQ Jackfruit Tacos with extra cilantro and serve with lime wedges on the side. The lime adds a zesty finish that cuts through the richness of the barbecue.

Troubleshooting Tip: Out of fresh cilantro? Chopped green onions or a dash of hot sauce can also elevate the flavor.

7. Taco Time Delight:

Dive into the flavor fiesta of your BBQ Jackfruit Tacos. Each bite is a symphony of smoky, tangy, and savory goodness. Don't forget to squeeze that lime for an extra burst of freshness.

Troubleshooting Tip: Taco overload? A napkin roll at the base prevents spillage.

Key Takeaway:

BBQ Jackfruit Tacos prove that plant-based eating can be both adventurous and comforting. So, gather 'round the taco table, savor the creative fusion of flavors, and let your taste buds dance in delight. It's not just a meal; it's a taco experience like no other.

Stuffed Bell Peppers with Wild Rice and Chickpeas

In this chapter of creative main courses, we're exploring two plant-powered delights that will elevate your dining experience, "Stuffed Bell Peppers with Wild Rice and Chickpeas" and "Sweet Potato and Black Bean Enchiladas."

Ingredients:

For the Stuffed Bell Peppers:
- 4 large bell peppers, halved and seeds removed
- 1 cup wild rice, cooked
- 1 can (15 oz) chickpeas, drained and rinsed
- 1 cup cherry tomatoes, diced
- 1/2 cup red onion, finely chopped
- 2 cloves garlic, minced
- 1 teaspoon cumin
- 1 teaspoon smoked paprika
- Salt and pepper to taste
- 1 cup tomato sauce
- Vegan cheese, shredded (optional for topping)
- Fresh parsley, chopped, for garnish

Instructions:

1. Bell Pepper Prep:

Preheat your oven to 375°F (190°C). Halve the bell peppers, removing the seeds and membranes. Place them in a baking dish.

Troubleshooting Tip: Wobbly peppers? Slice a tiny bit off the bottoms to create stability.

2. Rice and Chickpea Ensemble:

In a bowl, combine cooked wild rice, chickpeas, diced cherry tomatoes, chopped red onion, minced garlic, cumin, smoked paprika, salt, and pepper. Mix well – this is the flavorful ensemble for your stuffed peppers.

Troubleshooting Tip: Too dry? A drizzle of olive oil or a splash of vegetable broth adds moisture.

3. Stuff and Nestle:

Spoon the rice and chickpea mixture into each bell pepper half. Nestle them snugly into the baking dish.

Troubleshooting Tip: Overstuffing? Press the filling down gently to create a compact, delicious mound.

4. Saucy Drizzle:

Pour tomato sauce over the stuffed peppers, ensuring each one gets a saucy drizzle. This tomato bath adds that classic savory touch.

Troubleshooting Tip: Sauce too thin? Mix in a tablespoon of tomato paste for extra thickness.

5. Cheesy Crown (Optional):

If you're feeling cheesy, sprinkle vegan cheese over the stuffed peppers. This optional step adds a melty, gooey crown to your capsicum creation.

Troubleshooting Tip: Cheese not melting? Pop it under the broiler for a quick golden finish.

6. Bake and Garnish:

Bake in the preheated oven for about 25-30 minutes or until the peppers are tender. Once out of the oven, sprinkle fresh chopped parsley over the stuffed peppers for a burst of color and freshness.

Troubleshooting Tip: Peppers not tender? Cover with foil and bake a bit longer.

7. Serve and Enjoy:

Plate your Stuffed Bell Peppers with Wild Rice and Chickpeas, and dive into the symphony of flavors. Each bite is a harmonious blend of smoky, hearty goodness.

Troubleshooting Tip: Leftovers? These stuffed peppers make for a delicious next-day lunch.

Key Takeaway:

Stuffed Bell Peppers with Wild Rice and Chickpeas showcase that plant-based meals can be both wholesome and delicious. So, savor the textures, enjoy the medley of flavors, and relish in the joy of a creatively crafted dish.

Sweet Potato and Black Bean Enchiladas

Ingredients:

For the Enchilada Filling:
- 2 large sweet potatoes, peeled and diced
- 1 can (15 oz) black beans, drained and rinsed
- 1 red bell pepper, diced
- 1 red onion, finely chopped
- 2 cloves garlic, minced
- 1 teaspoon ground cumin
- 1 teaspoon chili powder
- Salt and pepper to taste
- 1 cup corn kernels (fresh, frozen, or canned)
- 1/4 cup fresh cilantro, chopped
- Juice of 1 lime

For the Enchilada Sauce:
- 2 cups tomato sauce
- 1 teaspoon ground cumin
- 1 teaspoon chili powder
- 1/2 teaspoon garlic powder
- Salt and pepper to taste

For Assembling:
- 8 large flour tortillas
- Vegan cheese, shredded (optional for topping)
- Fresh cilantro, chopped, for garnish

- Avocado slices, for serving

Instructions:

1. Sweet Potato Fiesta:

Preheat your oven to 375°F (190°C). In a baking dish, toss diced sweet potatoes with olive oil, salt, and pepper. Roast until they're tender and slightly caramelized.

Troubleshooting Tip: Roasting too slow? Increase the oven temperature for a quicker cook.

2. Filling Fiesta:

In a large bowl, combine roasted sweet potatoes, black beans, diced red bell pepper, finely chopped red onion, minced garlic, ground cumin, chili powder, salt, pepper, corn kernels, chopped cilantro, and lime juice. Mix this vibrant filling, it's a fiesta in a bowl.

Troubleshooting Tip: Cilantro aversion? Fresh parsley can bring a green touch without the cilantro flavor.

3. Saucy Sensation:

In a separate bowl, whisk together tomato sauce, ground cumin, chili powder, garlic powder, salt, and pepper. This is your zesty enchilada sauce, a sensation for your taste buds.

Troubleshooting Tip: Sauce too thick? Add a bit of water to reach a pourable consistency.

4. Roll and Assemble:

Spoon the filling onto each flour tortilla, roll it up, and place it seam side down in a baking dish. Repeat until all your enchiladas are snugly rolled.

Troubleshooting Tip: Tortillas cracking? Warm them slightly in the microwave or on the stovetop for flexibility.

5. Sauce and Cheesy Crown:

Pour the zesty enchilada sauce over the rolled beauties. If you're feeling cheesy, sprinkle vegan cheese on top for that melty finish.

Troubleshooting Tip: Sauce not spreading evenly? Use the back of a spoon to distribute it.

6. Bake to Perfection:

Bake in the preheated oven for about 20-25 minutes or until the enchiladas are heated through, and the edges are golden and bubbly.

Troubleshooting Tip: Cheese not melting? Broil for a minute for that golden touch.

7. Garnish and Serve:

Garnish your Sweet Potato and Black Bean Enchiladas with chopped fresh cilantro and serve with slices of ripe avocado on the side.

Troubleshooting Tip: Avocado not ripe? A squeeze of lime adds that zesty kick.

8. Enjoy the Southwestern Fiesta:

Plate your enchiladas, and dive into the Southwestern fiesta of flavors. Each bite is a journey through the heartiness of sweet potatoes, the earthiness of black beans, and the zesty embrace of enchilada sauce.

Troubleshooting Tip: Too many enchiladas? They freeze well for future quick meals.

Key Takeaway:

Sweet Potato and Black Bean Enchiladas bring a taste of the Southwest to your table, proving that plant-based meals can be a vibrant celebration of flavors. So, roll up those tortillas, embrace the spicy kick, and revel in the joy of a fiesta on your plate.

Chapter 7

Decadent Desserts

Rich Chocolate Avocado Mousse

As we embark on the sweet journey of decadent desserts, get ready to indulge in a symphony of flavors that redefine the meaning of sweet endings. In this chapter, our spotlight shines on "Rich Chocolate Avocado Mousse" a luscious creation that combines velvety richness with the goodness of avocados.

Ingredients:
- 3 ripe avocados, peeled and pitted
- 1/2 cup unsweetened cocoa powder
- 1/2 cup maple syrup or agave nectar
- 1/4 cup almond milk (or any plant-based milk)
- 1 teaspoon vanilla extract
- A pinch of salt
- Vegan whipped cream and chocolate shavings for garnish (optional)

Instructions:

1. Avocado Elegance:

Start by scooping out the ripe avocados into a blender or food processor. The creamy texture of avocados is the secret to achieving that luxurious mousse consistency.

Troubleshooting Tip: Avocados not ripe? Wait until they yield slightly to gentle pressure.

2. Cocoa Bliss:

Add unsweetened cocoa powder to the avocados. This is where the magic happens, the deep, rich chocolate flavor that will elevate your mousse to decadent heights.

Troubleshooting Tip: Cocoa lumps? Sift it before blending for a smoother texture.

3. Sweet Symphony:

Pour in the maple syrup or agave nectar, adding the perfect level of sweetness. Adjust the amount to suit your taste preferences.

Troubleshooting Tip: Too sweet or not sweet enough? Taste and adjust as needed.

4. Liquid Harmony:

Introduce almond milk (or your preferred plant-based milk) into the mix. This not only adds a touch of creaminess but also helps in achieving that silky smooth texture.

Troubleshooting Tip: Mousse too thick? Add a splash more almond milk for the desired consistency.

5. Vanilla Euphoria:

Enhance the flavor profile with a teaspoon of vanilla extract. The vanilla notes will complement the chocolatey richness, creating a harmonious blend.

Troubleshooting Tip: No vanilla extract? Vanilla bean paste or the seeds from a vanilla bean work beautifully.

6. Salt Essence:

Add a pinch of salt to intensify the chocolate flavor. This subtle addition balances the sweetness and enhances the overall taste.

Troubleshooting Tip: Too salty? Counteract with a bit more sweetener.

7. Blend to Perfection:

Blend all the ingredients until the mixture is velvety smooth. Pause and scrape down the sides if needed.

Witness the transformation from simple ingredients to a decadent chocolate masterpiece.

Troubleshooting Tip: Avocado bits? Keep blending until the mousse is uniformly smooth.

8. Chill and Set:

Transfer the chocolate avocado mousse to individual serving bowls or glasses. Allow it to chill in the refrigerator for at least 2 hours, allowing the flavors to meld and the mousse to set.

Troubleshooting Tip: Impatient? Pop it in the freezer for a quick chill, but don't forget to check periodically.

9. Garnish and Serve:

When ready to serve, top the mousse with a dollop of vegan whipped cream and a sprinkle of chocolate shavings if you're feeling extra indulgent.

Troubleshooting Tip: Whipped cream not holding? Ensure it's well chilled before whipping.

10. Savor the Decadence:

Dive into the richness of your Rich Chocolate Avocado Mousse. Each spoonful is a celebration of velvety smoothness, chocolatey bliss, and the surprising goodness of avocados.

Troubleshooting Tip: Mousse too firm? Let it sit at room temperature for a few minutes before serving.

Key Takeaway:
Rich Chocolate Avocado Mousse is a testament to the fact that decadent desserts can be both indulgent and health-conscious. So, savor the velvety goodness, delight in the chocolatey symphony, and relish the guilt-free pleasure of a dessert that transcends the ordinary.

Vegan Cheesecake with Berry Compote

In this chapter of decadent desserts, prepare to satisfy your sweet cravings with two plant-powered delights, "Vegan Cheesecake with Berry Compote" and "Almond Butter Banana Bread."

Ingredients:

For the Cheesecake:
- 2 cups raw cashews, soaked overnight
- 1 cup coconut cream
- 1/2 cup coconut oil, melted
- 1/2 cup maple syrup or agave nectar
- 1/4 cup lemon juice
- 1 teaspoon vanilla extract
- A pinch of salt

For the Berry Compote:
- 2 cups mixed berries (strawberries, blueberries, raspberries)
- 1/4 cup maple syrup or agave nectar
- 1 tablespoon lemon juice
- Zest of 1 lemon

For the Crust:
- 1 cup almond flour
- 1/4 cup coconut oil, melted

- 2 tablespoons maple syrup or agave nectar
- A pinch of salt

Instructions:

1. Crust Creation:

In a bowl, combine almond flour, melted coconut oil, maple syrup, and a pinch of salt. Press this mixture into the base of a springform pan, creating the perfect foundation for your cheesecake.

Troubleshooting Tip: Crust too dry? Add a bit more melted coconut oil for moisture.

2. Cashew Cream Bliss:

In a blender, combine soaked cashews, coconut cream, melted coconut oil, maple syrup, lemon juice, vanilla extract, and a pinch of salt. Blend until you achieve a silky smooth consistency, the essence of your creamy vegan cheesecake.

Troubleshooting Tip: Cashew cream too thick? Add a splash of coconut cream to reach the desired creaminess.

3. Pour and Set:

Pour the cashew cream over the prepared crust in the springform pan. Smooth the top with a spatula for an even surface. Allow the cheesecake to set in the freezer for at least 4 hours or overnight.

Troubleshooting Tip: Cheesecake not setting? Ensure it's in the coldest part of your freezer.

4. Berry Compote Magic:

In a saucepan, combine mixed berries, maple syrup, lemon juice, and lemon zest. Simmer over low heat until the berries break down and the mixture thickens. Let it cool before generously drizzling over the chilled cheesecake.

Troubleshooting Tip: Compote too runny? Simmer a bit longer to reach your desired thickness.

5. Slice and Serve:

Once the cheesecake has set, carefully remove it from the springform pan. Slice into decadent portions and serve each piece with a generous spoonful of the berry compote.

Troubleshooting Tip: Difficulty slicing? Dip your knife in hot water for smoother cuts.

6. Garnish and Enjoy:

Garnish your Vegan Cheesecake with Berry Compote with extra fresh berries or a sprinkle of mint leaves for a burst of color. Each bite is a symphony of creamy richness and fruity sweetness.

Troubleshooting Tip: Out of fresh berries? A dusting of powdered sugar can add a touch of elegance.

7. Delight in Creamy Sweetness:

Delight in the velvety texture of your Vegan Cheesecake with Berry Compote. Every forkful is a celebration of plant-based indulgence, proving that dessert can be both luxurious and compassionate.

Troubleshooting Tip: Leftovers? Store in the freezer for a delicious frozen treat.

Key Takeaway:

Vegan Cheesecake with Berry Compote is a dessert masterpiece that showcases the magic of plant-based ingredients. So, savor the creamy bliss, enjoy the burst of berry sweetness, and revel in the joy of a dessert that's both decadent and dairy-free.

Almond Butter Banana Bread

Ingredients:

- 3 ripe bananas, mashed
- 1/2 cup almond butter
- 1/4 cup coconut oil, melted
- 1/2 cup coconut sugar
- 1 flax egg (1 tablespoon flaxseed meal + 3 tablespoons water)
- 1 teaspoon vanilla extract
- 1 3/4 cups almond flour
- 1/2 cup oat flour
- 1 teaspoon baking soda
- 1/2 teaspoon cinnamon
- A pinch of salt
- 1/2 cup chopped almonds for topping (optional)

Instructions:

1. Banana Bliss:

Preheat your oven to 350°F (175°C). In a bowl, mash the ripe bananas until smooth. This forms the sweet and moist base of your almond butter banana bread.

Troubleshooting Tip: Bananas not ripe enough? Wait until they develop brown spots for maximum sweetness.

2. Nutty Harmony:

Add almond butter, melted coconut oil, coconut sugar, flax egg, and vanilla extract to the mashed bananas. Mix until well combined, creating a nutty and flavorful blend.

Troubleshooting Tip: Almond butter too thick? Gently warm it for easier mixing.

3. Flour Fusion:

In a separate bowl, combine almond flour, oat flour, baking soda, cinnamon, and a pinch of salt. Gradually fold this dry mixture into the wet ingredients until a smooth batter forms.

Troubleshooting Tip: Batter too dry? Add a splash of almond milk for moisture.

4. Bake and Rise:

Pour the batter into a greased or parchment-lined loaf pan. Spread it evenly and tap the pan on the counter to release any air bubbles. Optionally, sprinkle chopped almonds on top for a delightful crunch.

Troubleshooting Tip: Loaf sinking in the middle? Check the freshness of your baking soda.

5. Oven Love:

Bake in the preheated oven for approximately 45-50 minutes or until a toothpick inserted into the center comes out clean. The aroma wafting through your kitchen is a delicious promise.

Troubleshooting Tip: Top browning too quickly? Tent the loaf with foil to prevent over-browning.

6. Cool and Slice:

Allow the almond butter banana bread to cool in the pan for about 15 minutes before transferring it to a wire rack to cool completely. This patience ensures a perfectly moist and sliceable bread.

Troubleshooting Tip: Slicing too crumbly? Chill the bread before slicing for cleaner cuts.

7. Slice and Enjoy:

Once cooled, slice your almond butter banana bread into thick, tempting slices. Serve it as is or with a smear of additional almond butter for an extra nutty touch.

Troubleshooting Tip: Bread too dense? Ensure your flax egg is well mixed and your baking soda is fresh.

8. Nourish with Nutty Goodness:

Nourish your senses with the nutty goodness of your Almond Butter Banana Bread. Each bite is a comforting blend of sweet bananas, rich almond butter, and the warm embrace of cinnamon.

Troubleshooting Tip: Storing leftovers? Wrap slices in parchment paper before storing to maintain freshness.

Key Takeaway:

Almond Butter Banana Bread is a delightful twist on a classic favorite, showcasing the heartwarming combination of bananas and nutty almond butter. So, savor the nutty notes, relish the moist texture, and bask in the joy of a comforting treat that's both wholesome and indulgent.

Chapter 8

Beverages and Smoothies

Green Goddess Detox Smoothie

Welcome to the revitalizing world of Chapter 8, where we explore the refreshing realm of beverages and smoothies. In this chapter, our focus is on the "Green Goddess Detox Smoothie" a vibrant concoction that not only tantalizes your taste buds but also gives your body a nourishing boost.

Ingredients:
- 1 cup kale leaves, stems removed
- 1 cup spinach leaves
- 1/2 cucumber, peeled and sliced
- 1 green apple, cored and chopped
- 1/2 lemon, juiced
- 1/2 inch fresh ginger, peeled
- 1 cup coconut water
- 1 tablespoon chia seeds (optional for added texture)
- Ice cubes (optional for a chilled smoothie)

Instructions:

1. Green Symphony Begins:
Gather your green warriors, kale, spinach, cucumber, and green apple. These nutrient-packed ingredients form the base of your Green Goddess Detox Smoothie.

Troubleshooting Tip: Greens too bitter? Adjust the balance by adding a bit more apple or a squeeze of lemon.

2. Citrus Zing:
Squeeze the juice of half a lemon into the mix. This not only adds a refreshing citrus zing but also enhances the body's ability to absorb the nutrients from the greens.

Troubleshooting Tip: Lemon too tart? Adjust by adding a touch of sweetness from a ripe banana or a splash of apple juice.

3. Ginger Kick:
Grate or finely chop the fresh ginger. This ingredient brings a delightful kick to your smoothie while contributing its anti-inflammatory and digestive benefits.

Troubleshooting Tip: Ginger too strong? Start with a smaller amount and adjust according to your preference.

4. Cucumber Coolness:

Peel and slice half a cucumber, introducing a cool and hydrating element to your smoothie. Cucumber also adds a subtle sweetness without overpowering the greens.

Troubleshooting Tip: Smoothie too thick? Add a bit more coconut water for a lighter consistency.

5. Apple Freshness:

Core and chop a green apple, adding a touch of natural sweetness to balance the earthiness of the greens. The apple also contributes fiber for a satisfying texture.

Troubleshooting Tip: Apple not sweet enough? Try a different variety or add a drizzle of honey.

6. Leafy Greens Dance:

Toss in the kale and spinach leaves, packed with vitamins and minerals. These leafy greens are the backbone of your Green Goddess, offering a nutrient-rich foundation.

Troubleshooting Tip: Blender struggling? Add the greens gradually and blend in stages.

7. Chia Seeds (Optional):

For those who enjoy a bit of texture, add chia seeds to the mix. These tiny powerhouses are rich in fiber and omega-3 fatty acids, providing an extra nutritional boost.

Troubleshooting Tip: Chia seeds absorbing too much liquid? Let the smoothie sit for a few minutes and stir before drinking.

8. Coconut Water Hydration:

Pour in the coconut water, infusing your smoothie with natural electrolytes and hydration. This tropical addition also complements the green flavors with a touch of sweetness.

Troubleshooting Tip: Coconut water too sweet? Opt for an unsweetened variety or adjust the quantity.

9. Blitz into Bliss:

Fire up your blender and watch the vibrant ingredients transform into a silky green elixir. Blend until the mixture is smooth, and the green hues are evenly distributed.

Troubleshooting Tip: Smoothie too thick? Gradually add more liquid until you reach your desired consistency.

10. Chill and Serve:

If you prefer a chilled experience, toss in some ice cubes before giving the final blend. Pour your Green Goddess Detox Smoothie into a glass and marvel at the verdant beauty.

Troubleshooting Tip: Ice too noisy? Use frozen fruits or chill the ingredients beforehand.

11. Garnish and Sip:

Garnish your smoothie with a slice of cucumber or a sprinkle of chia seeds for a touch of elegance. Sip and relish the rejuvenating flavors that dance on your palate.

Troubleshooting Tip: Smoothie not sweet enough? A drizzle of honey or a ripe banana in the mix can enhance sweetness.

12. Nourish Your Body:

Nourish your body with the Green Goddess Detox Smoothie, a liquid infusion of vitamins, minerals, and antioxidants. Let each sip be a celebration of wellness and the vibrant energy of green goodness.

Troubleshooting Tip: New to green smoothies? Start with milder greens like baby spinach and gradually incorporate heartier greens like kale.

Key Takeaway:
The Green Goddess Detox Smoothie is a testament to the fact that a nutrient-packed beverage can be both delicious and revitalizing. So, sip your way to radiance, embrace the green vitality, and revel in the joy of a smoothie that nourishes from the inside out. Cheers to vibrant health and a refreshed spirit!

Refreshing Mint-Lime Cooler

Prepare to quench your thirst and revitalize your senses with two delightful creations in the beverage wonderland, the "Refreshing Mint-Lime Cooler" and the "Energizing Matcha Latte."

Ingredients:

- 1 cup fresh mint leaves
- Juice of 3 limes
- 2 tablespoons honey or agave nectar
- 4 cups cold sparkling water
- Ice cubes
- Lime slices and mint sprigs for garnish

Instructions:

1. Minty Freshness:

Begin by muddling fresh mint leaves in a glass. This releases the aromatic oils and sets the stage for a truly refreshing experience.

Troubleshooting Tip: Mint too strong? Adjust the quantity based on your preference.

2. Zesty Lime Infusion:

Squeeze the juice of three limes into the glass. The zesty lime infusion complements the mint, creating a lively combination of citrusy and herbal notes.

Troubleshooting Tip: Lime too tart? Balance it with a bit more honey or agave nectar.

3. Sweet Nectar:

Add honey or agave nectar to the mix, sweetening the concoction to your liking. Stir well to ensure the sweetness is evenly distributed.

Troubleshooting Tip: Honey not dissolving? Warm it slightly before adding to ease the mixing process.

4. Sparkling Fizz:

Pour cold sparkling water into the glass, creating a fizzy effervescence that lifts the flavors of mint and lime. This effervescent twist adds a playful element to your cooler.

Troubleshooting Tip: Fizz too strong? Stir gently to reduce the bubbles.

5. Ice Wonderland:

Drop in ice cubes, turning your mint-lime concoction into a chilly wonderland. The ice not only cools the drink but enhances the overall experience.

Troubleshooting Tip: Ice melting too quickly? Use larger ice cubes or consider freezing a portion of the sparkling water into ice cubes.

6. Garnish Galore:

Elevate the visual appeal by garnishing your mint-lime cooler with lime slices and a sprig of fresh mint. This not only looks enticing but also adds a burst of fragrance with each sip.

Troubleshooting Tip: Mint leaves turning brown? Store them properly, wrapped in a damp paper towel in the refrigerator.

7. Sip and Enjoy:

Take a sip of your Refreshing Mint-Lime Cooler and let the combination of minty coolness and zesty lime tickle your taste buds. This is the ultimate elixir for beating the heat and staying revitalized.

Troubleshooting Tip: Not refreshing enough? Adjust the mint and lime quantities for a stronger flavor.

Key Takeaway:

The Refreshing Mint-Lime Cooler is a celebration of summer in a glass, proving that simple ingredients can create a symphony of flavors. So, sip, savor, and let the mint-lime magic transport you to a state of refreshing bliss.

Energizing Matcha Latte

Ingredients:

- 1 teaspoon matcha powder
- 1 cup unsweetened almond milk (or any plant-based milk)
- 1-2 tablespoons maple syrup or sweetener of choice
- Hot water (not boiling)
- Optional: Vanilla extract or vanilla-flavored plant milk
- Optional: Whisked coconut cream for topping

Instructions:

1. Matcha Magic Unleashed:

Begin by sifting matcha powder into a bowl. Sifting ensures a smooth and lump-free matcha base for your latte.

Troubleshooting Tip: Matcha too clumpy? Whisk it thoroughly or use a fine-mesh strainer for sifting.

2. Hot Water Elixir:

Pour a small amount of hot water (not boiling) into the bowl with the sifted matcha. Whisk the mixture vigorously using a bamboo matcha whisk or a small whisk until a smooth, vibrant green paste forms.

Troubleshooting Tip: Matcha paste too thick? Gradually add more hot water and whisk until the desired consistency is reached.

3. Sweet Symphony:

In a separate saucepan, heat almond milk until it's warm but not boiling. Add the warm almond milk to the matcha paste, creating a velvety green elixir.

Troubleshooting Tip: Milk curdling? Ensure your milk is not too hot, and gradually incorporate it into the matcha.

4. Sweeten the Deal:

Add maple syrup or your sweetener of choice to the matcha latte, adjusting the sweetness to your preference. Stir well to ensure even sweetness throughout.

Troubleshooting Tip: Latte not sweet enough? Add a bit more sweetener or experiment with flavored syrups.

5. Optional Flavor Enhancements:

For an extra flavor kick, add a few drops of vanilla extract or use vanilla-flavored plant milk. This subtle addition enhances the overall taste of your matcha latte.

Troubleshooting Tip: Vanilla overpowering? Start with a small amount and adjust to taste.

6. Whisk to Perfection:

Whisk the matcha latte one more time to create a frothy layer on top. The froth adds a delightful texture and elevates the visual appeal.

Troubleshooting Tip: No frother or whisk? Shake the latte vigorously in a sealed container or use an electric blender.

7. Pour and Top:

Pour your energizing matcha latte into a mug, marveling at its vibrant green hue. If you desire an extra indulgence, top it off with whisked coconut cream for a luxurious finishing touch.

Troubleshooting Tip: Latte too thin? Increase the matcha powder for a bolder flavor.

8. Sip and Invigorate:

Take a sip of your Energizing Matcha Latte and feel the wave of green energy invigorating your senses. The earthy notes of matcha, combined with the creamy almond milk, make every sip a moment of pure bliss.

Troubleshooting Tip: Matcha settling at the bottom? Give your latte a gentle stir before each sip.

Key Takeaway:
The Energizing Matcha Latte is not just a drink; it's a revitalizing experience that combines the power of matcha with the comforting creaminess of almond milk. So, sip, savor, and let the green magic recharge your body and mind. Cheers to the invigorating world of matcha!

Chapter 9

Meal Planning and Tips

Weekly Vegan Meal Planner

As we dive into Chapter 9, we embark on a journey that goes beyond individual recipes, a journey into the art and science of meal planning. This chapter is not just about cooking; it's about crafting a seamless, delicious, and sustainable vegan culinary experience. Let's explore "Weekly Vegan Meal Planner," "Budget-Friendly Vegan Cooking," and "Quick and Easy Weeknight Dinners."

Creating a weekly vegan meal plan is like composing a symphony of flavors that dance through the week. It's about balance, variety, and ensuring every meal is a delight for your taste buds and a nourishment for your body.

Guiding Principles for a Weekly Vegan Meal Plan:

1. Diverse Nutritional Palette:
Ensure your meals span a spectrum of colors, textures, and nutrients. Aim to incorporate a variety of fruits,

vegetables, grains, legumes, and plant-based proteins throughout the week.

2. Balance of Macronutrients:

Strike a balance between carbohydrates, proteins, and healthy fats. This not only keeps your energy levels steady but also ensures your body receives a well-rounded nutritional profile.

3. Meal Prep Efficiency:

Plan meals that allow for some overlap in ingredients, making meal prep more efficient. For example, if you're chopping vegetables for a salad, consider using the same veggies for a stir-fry later in the week.

4. Seasonal and Local:

Embrace seasonal and local produce for freshness and flavor. Not only does this support local farmers, but it also adds a dynamic quality to your meals based on what's available.

5. Mindful Portions:

Consider portion sizes to prevent overbuying and reduce food waste. Leftovers can be repurposed creatively or enjoyed as quick and convenient lunches.

6. Flexibility and Adaptability:
Be flexible with your plan. Life happens, and sometimes plans change. Having a flexible attitude allows you to adapt and still enjoy delicious meals.

Example Weekly Vegan Meal Planner:

Monday:
Breakfast: Avocado Toast with Cherry Tomatoes
Lunch: Quinoa Salad with Mixed Vegetables and Chickpeas
Dinner: Lentil and Vegetable Stew with Brown Rice

Tuesday:
Breakfast: Berry Smoothie Bowl
Lunch: Sweet Potato and Black Bean Enchiladas
Dinner: Creamy Mushroom Alfredo Pasta

Wednesday:
Breakfast: Overnight Oats with Almond Milk and Fresh Fruit
Lunch: Caesar Salad with Cashew Caesar Dressing
Dinner: BBQ Jackfruit Tacos with Cabbage Slaw

Thursday:
Breakfast: Vegan Banana Pancakes with Maple Syrup
Lunch: Southwestern Black Bean Salad

Dinner: Classic Tomato Basil Soup with Whole Grain Bread

Friday:
Breakfast: Chia Seed Pudding with Mango
Lunch: Quinoa and Roasted Vegetable Salad
Dinner: Eggplant Parmesan with Cashew Cheese

Saturday:
Breakfast: Tofu Scramble with Spinach and Tomatoes
Lunch: Coconut Curry Butternut Squash Soup
Dinner: Stuffed Bell Peppers with Wild Rice and Chickpeas

Sunday:
Breakfast: Vegan Breakfast Burritos with Salsa
Lunch: Creamy Broccoli and Potato Soup
Dinner: Spaghetti Bolognese with Lentil Meatballs

Key Takeaway:
A Weekly Vegan Meal Planner is your roadmap to a week filled with delightful, nutritious, and diverse plant-based meals. It not only streamlines your cooking process but also ensures that each day is a culinary adventure.

Budget-Friendly Vegan Cooking

Cooking on a budget doesn't mean compromising on flavor or nutrition. It's about making savvy choices, utilizing affordable ingredients, and maximizing your culinary creativity. Here are some tips for budget-friendly vegan cooking:

Tips for Budget-Friendly Vegan Cooking:

1. Embrace Staple Ingredients:
Build your pantry around budget-friendly staples like rice, lentils, beans, oats, and pasta. These ingredients form the foundation for countless affordable and nutritious meals.

2. Buy in Bulk:
Purchase pantry staples in bulk to save money in the long run. Items like grains, legumes, and nuts often have a lower price per unit when bought in larger quantities.

3. Seasonal and Local Produce:
Opt for seasonal and local produce, as they tend to be more budget-friendly and flavorful. Visit local farmers' markets or explore discounted sections in grocery stores for deals on fresh produce.

4. Frozen Fruits and Vegetables:

Frozen fruits and vegetables are not only convenient but also often more affordable than fresh. They have a longer shelf life, making them a practical choice for budget-conscious cooking.

5. DIY Plant-Based Proteins:

Experiment with making your own plant-based protein sources, like cooking dried beans or preparing tofu at home. It's often more economical than purchasing pre-packaged alternatives.

6. Meal Prep and Batch Cooking:

Plan and prepare meals in batches. This not only saves time but also allows you to take advantage of sales and discounts when buying ingredients in larger quantities.

7. Repurpose Leftovers:

Get creative with leftovers to avoid food waste. For example, use last night's roasted vegetables in a wrap or stir-fry, or repurpose a grain dish into a hearty salad.

8. Limit Specialty Ingredients:

While specialty vegan products can be tempting, they can also be expensive. Limit the use of specialty items and focus on whole, unprocessed foods for a budget-friendly approach.

Budget-Friendly Vegan Recipe: Lentil and Vegetable Stir-Fry

Ingredients:
- 1 cup dried green lentils
- 2 cups mixed vegetables (carrots, bell peppers, broccoli)
- 1 onion, sliced
- 3 cloves garlic, minced
- 1 tablespoon soy sauce
- 1 tablespoon maple syrup
- 1 teaspoon sesame oil
- Cooked rice or noodles for serving

Instructions:
1. Cook the green lentils according to the package instructions. Drain and set aside.
2. In a large pan or wok, sauté the sliced onion and minced garlic until fragrant.
3. Add the mixed vegetables to the pan and stir-fry until they are tender-crisp.
4. Incorporate the cooked lentils into the vegetable mixture, combining them evenly.
5. In a small bowl, whisk together soy sauce, maple syrup, and sesame oil. Pour the sauce over the stir-fry and toss to coat.
6. Continue cooking for a few more minutes until the flavors meld and the stir-fry is heated through.

7. Serve the lentil and vegetable stir-fry over cooked rice or noodles.

Key Takeaway:
Budget-friendly vegan cooking is about making mindful choices, utilizing cost-effective ingredients, and embracing the creativity that comes with cooking on a budget. With these tips, you can enjoy delicious and nutritious plant-based meals without breaking the bank.

Quick and Easy Weeknight Dinners

In the hustle and bustle of daily life, quick and easy weeknight dinners become the saving grace for busy individuals and families. These meals are not only efficient but also deliver on flavor and nutrition. Here are some tips for mastering the art of quick and easy weeknight dinners:

Tips for Quick and Easy Weeknight Dinners:

1. Prep Ingredients in Advance:
Take advantage of downtime, such as the weekend, to prep and chop ingredients for the upcoming week. Having prepped veggies, cooked grains, and marinated proteins on hand accelerates the cooking process.

2. One-Pan Wonders:
Opt for one-pan or one-pot meals that minimize cleanup and streamline the cooking process. Sheet pan dinners, stir-fries, and casseroles are excellent choices for quick and easy preparation.

3. Batch Cook and Freeze:
Prepare larger quantities of your favorite recipes when time allows and freeze individual portions. This way, you'll always have a ready-made meal on hand for busy evenings.

4. Utilize Convenience Ingredients:

Leverage convenience ingredients like pre-cut vegetables, canned beans, and pre-cooked grains to expedite the cooking process. These items can be time-savers without compromising on nutrition.

5. Quick Cooking Methods:

Explore quick cooking methods such as sautéing, stir-frying, and grilling. These methods allow you to have a hot and flavorful meal on the table in minimal time.

6. 30-Minute Recipes:

Build a repertoire of go-to recipes that can be prepared in 30 minutes or less. These recipes are invaluable for those evenings when time is of the essence.

7. Simple Flavor Boosters:

Enhance the flavor of your dishes with simple and quick flavor boosters like fresh herbs, citrus zest, or a drizzle of flavored oils. These additions can elevate the taste without adding complexity.

8. No-Cook Options:

Embrace no-cook options on particularly hectic nights. This could include assembling hearty salads, wraps, or sandwiches using pre-prepped ingredients.

Quick and Easy Weeknight Dinner Recipe: Chickpea and Vegetable Stir-Fry

Ingredients:
- 1 can chickpeas, drained and rinsed
- 2 cups mixed vegetables (bell peppers, snap peas, carrots)
- 1 tablespoon vegetable oil
- 2 tablespoons soy sauce
- 1 tablespoon rice vinegar
- 1 teaspoon sesame oil
- 1 teaspoon grated ginger
- 2 cloves garlic, minced
- Cooked rice or noodles for serving

Instructions:
1. Heat vegetable oil in a large pan or wok over medium-high heat.
2. Add mixed vegetables to the pan and stir-fry until they are tender-crisp.
3. Incorporate drained chickpeas into the vegetable mixture, allowing them to heat through.
4. In a small bowl, whisk together soy sauce, rice vinegar, sesame oil, grated ginger, and minced garlic.
5. Pour the sauce over the stir-fry and toss to coat evenly. Cook for an additional 2-3 minutes.
6. Serve the chickpea and vegetable stir-fry over cooked rice or noodles.

Key Takeaway:
Quick and easy weeknight dinners are a testament to the notion that delicious and nutritious meals can be prepared in a short amount of time. With efficient strategies and simple recipes, you can conquer weeknight dinners with ease, making every meal a stress-free culinary delight.

Conclusion

As we bring our culinary journey to a close, it's not just about concluding a collection of recipes; it's about savoring the essence of creating comfort in every bite. In "How to Make Delicious Vegan Comfort Food Recipes: Creative Plant-Based Takes on Classic Crave-Worthy Meals," we've explored the art of transforming familiar favorites into plant-powered delights.

From the aromatic kitchens filled with the scent of coconut curry butternut squash soup to the joyous gatherings over BBQ jackfruit tacos, each recipe has been a chapter in the story of crafting comfort through plant-based creativity. It's not just about the ingredients; it's about the experience, the joy, and the connection we create with our food.

Through the laughter shared over a bowl of lentil and vegetable stew or the quiet moments relishing a slice of almond butter banana bread, we've woven a tapestry of flavors that transcend the plate. Vegan comfort food isn't just about dietary choices; it's a celebration of culinary innovation, a testament to the incredible versatility of plant-based ingredients, and a journey into the heart of what makes a meal truly satisfying.

As you embark on your own adventures in the kitchen, armed with the knowledge of essential ingredients, efficient cooking tips, and a repertoire of mouthwatering recipes, remember that each dish is an opportunity to infuse comfort and joy into your life and the lives of those you share it with.

So, whether you're simmering a pot of classic tomato basil soup, whipping up a quick and budget-friendly lentil stir-fry, or indulging in the decadence of rich chocolate avocado mousse, know that you're not just following recipes, you're creating moments of warmth and connection through the language of food.

As the pages of this cookbook close, may the aroma of your culinary creations linger in your memories, and may the flavors continue to dance on your taste buds. "How to Make Delicious Vegan Comfort Food Recipes" isn't just a guide; it's an invitation to infuse your kitchen with creativity, your meals with love, and your life with the joy of savoring every delicious moment.

Here's to a future filled with plant-powered comfort, culinary exploration, and the enduring joy of sharing a table laden with delicious vegan creations. Cheers to the journey, the flavors, and the boundless comfort found in each and every bite.

www.ingramcontent.com/pod-product-compliance
Lightning Source LLC
Chambersburg PA
CBHW070900260726
48661CB00004B/1521